SELF-HEALTH FIX

SELF-HEALTH FIX

How to Stop Being a Forever Patient and
Start Taking Charge of Your Well-Being
PLUS Your Personal Health Rating Scale

Rosalind Ferry

Editor, Nina Shoroplova—ninashoroplova.ca
Book Interior and eBook Design, Amit Dey—amitdey2528@gmail.com
Publishing Consultant, Geoff Affleck—geoff@geoffaffleck.com

To my dearest mother, Pat, a wonderful nurse and listener who inspired me to overcome my health issues and taught me that we humans have more power to heal ourselves than we think.

Contents

Acknowledgements

I would like to thank my generous husband, Jon, and my wonderful son, Will, for encouraging me to write this book and helping me with editing and technical support. I could not have done this without you both.

Many thanks to Geoff Affleck, book entrepreneur extraordinaire, whose patience and skill guided me smoothly through the complex production and marketing process.

Thanks to Nina Shoroplova for her masterful editing, patience, and kindness.

And thanks to all the amazing patients I have had the pleasure of working with through the years. I have learned so much from you all, and hope your stories will help others find solutions to their health problems.

Thanks to the doctors and other health professionals who entrusted me with the care of their patients. And a special thanks to Anniken Chadwick, the physiotherapist who contributed a valuable chapter to this book.

My gratitude also goes to long-time friend Jane Morgan, a true warrior. Her story is an inspiration to us all.

Finally, I would like to acknowledge my beautiful, spirited grandchildren, Georgia and Julian, whose creative talents give me hope for a better, healthier world.

Preface

When it comes to their health, some patients seem to be *forever patients*. They never appear to recover fully or think that this is even possible.

They have lost faith in their body's ability to heal, and expect little from the health system . . . so little that they are content if it simply gives them a Band-Aid.

I vividly remember returning to work at a British Columbia hospital out-patient clinic and being shocked to see several patients I had treated seven years earlier—for the same conditions.

I thought then, as I do now, that many of them had been programmed to remain victims of their own low expectations.

My motivation in writing this book is a growing belief that we cannot depend on the overworked health system alone for an improvement in our well-being. We must learn to care for our own bodies and have a plan for keeping them in tip-top shape, just as we would our finances and friendships.

Instead, too many of us seem to believe that, because of bad luck or poor genetics, we are locked into a state of perpetual sub-par existence, supported by the medical system.

Many health professionals, too, appear content for this dependency to continue. Or at least they seem to feel they don't have the time to discuss the fullest possible range of treatment options, including those that put patients in charge of their own health.

My research for this book started with my own hands-on experience as a physiotherapist, treating a wide range of patients in both hospital and private practice in Britain and Canada for more than forty years.

My study mushroomed with the work for my book *The Posture Pain Fix*, a step-by-step guide to help people ease their neck, back, and other body-alignment problems. And I have supplemented that research with my reading on everything from homeopathy and holistic healing to Pilates, the Feldenkrais Method, and other physical fitness and therapy systems.

Self-care isn't a new concept. Greek philosopher Socrates stressed its importance in the fifth century BCE, and everyone from the Persian poet Rumi in the thirteenth century to British political theorist John Locke in the seventeenth century have continued to do so.

Today, doctors and health systems managers on the front lines in the battle against COVID-19 invoke self-care's efficacy.

As Washington, DC, internal medicine specialist Manisha Singal, MD, stated, "I make it a point to practise self-care. In fact, I make an appointment with myself. I spend this time to meditate and affirm three things that I'm grateful for that day."

I, too, make regular appointments with myself. And I hope this book will help encourage you to do so too.

Note: In the context of my having worked as a physiotherapist, I occasionally refer to myself as a *physio* and my practice as a *physio clinic.*

CHAPTER 1

Trusting Your Gut

A few years ago, I was going home from work after a busy day at my North Vancouver physiotherapy clinic. It was a ten-minute walk alongside a saltwater inlet ringed by mountains and forests. A man slowly drew up beside me in his truck, stopped, and said, "You'd better get in my vehicle . . . there's a bear on the street."

This middle-aged man was a stranger. I looked at him, thanked him, and told him I'd be okay. He drove off, leaving me to proceed with caution. And, sure enough, there was a black bear in the bushes beside the road.

I continued home calmly, but was ready to react. The bear continued on its way, too. Having grown up in Africa around wild animals, I believed I had the confidence to navigate around them with quiet, alert energy, knowing full well they could be unpredictable.

In other words, I made a split-second decision to take my chances with a bear rather than getting into an automobile with a man I knew nothing about. For some people, though, the decision might have been the exact opposite.

So, the question arises, whom do you really trust? Perhaps close friends and relatives. Or maybe just yourself. In which case, developing self-reliance skills is essential.

However, knowing when to rely on yourself and when it's best to seek professional medical help often is not a simple decision. People tend either to go to the doctor at the first tickle of the throat . . . or wait until they are in the middle of a stroke or heart attack. Mothers and wives will know what I'm talking about.

My son joined us for breakfast the other morning. It was a warm, humid day and he said he was feeling weak and very tired. My immediate reaction was "Oh, no, it's the coronavirus."

He felt hot, clammy, and tired. I took his temperature, and it was normal. He had no dry cough, no chest pain or trouble breathing, and no scratchy throat (all possible COVID-19 symptoms). This was a relief for us all.

Then, I remembered our son had gone on an intense, hour-long mountain-bike ride the previous evening. And he acknowledged he had been sweating a lot without taking in regular fluids.

I suggested he drink water, to which I added some salt. He drank three glasses slowly with the salt, relaxed for an hour and said, "I am feeling quite a bit better, thanks."

The moral of this story is for people to be aware, especially during this or any other pandemic, of any noticeable health changes. Then, they should look at the obvious stuff first . . . in this case the need to replenish lost fluids.

For example, California nutritionist Trudy Scott, author of the *Antianxiety Food Solution*, recommends drinking at least two quarts (64 fluid ounces) of water daily, and more if you are exercising.

In other words, try the simple, common-sense fixes first. Often, they are the best. Also, learn to trust in your own hard-earned experience dealing with life's possible dangers. Sometimes, you just have to trust your gut.

CHAPTER 2

My Personal Health Struggles

What are the important things in life? Friendships, certainly, and a passion for living is clearly key. But perhaps the most underrated aspect of our lives is our health.

Health is a gauge of how well we are doing and coping. It's also wonderful in its own right. People who brim with good health radiate those positive vibrations that make others want to be their friends so they can share their passions.

Healthy humans are generally well-adjusted people who are in balance with their minds, bodies, and the world around them. But being healthy requires constant attention and work.

I was a fairly healthy child, but suffered from many ear and throat infections . . . for which I was given multiple doses of antibiotics. These treatments affected the bacterial balance in my gut, and led to everything from anxiety to skin irritations.

In my teenage years, I started to develop skin problems, and suffered from bouts of urticaria (hives) whenever I became badly stressed.

My face would blow up as if it had been inflated by a bicycle pump. This would invariably happen when I flew home from boarding school in the UK to Kenya, my parents' home. I looked as if I had some dreadful, contagious condition, which proved highly embarrassing.

Doctors at my British school investigated me for tropical diseases, but the tests proved negative.

Eventually, one frustrated physician said, "Perhaps she is suffering from unrequited love." As a young, naïve teenager, I didn't even know what he was talking about.

My mother, a nurse, came to my rescue. She said, "Rosalind, you are going to have to sort this out yourself by telling yourself over and over again that your skin will get better. And it will."

I can't thank my mother enough for her wisdom and the lesson in mind-body control she gave me … long before so-called alternative medicine was in vogue. And to this day I no longer suffer from skin blow-ups.

However, I also inherited from my mother a condition called otosclerosis, or calcification of the stapes bone in the middle ear. It causes deafness. My mother had it in one of her ears; I had it in both.

My progressive hearing loss was accompanied by tinnitus, which generated an unrelenting stream of whirring noises. It was highly debilitating. Working as a physiotherapist and needing to hear my patients' concerns, I eventually had to wear a hearing aid.

Over the years, I had four surgeries on my left ear and various tubes to compensate for a badly scarred left eardrum. My eustachian tubes would always get plugged if I had a cold, leading to painful bouts of middle ear infection (*otitis media*) and ruptured eardrums.

One day at work in British Columbia, I remember starting a cold. Later that evening, I could hear nothing, not even the shower running. I was devastated, and believed I might have to give up my physiotherapy practice.

I saw my ear, nose, and throat doctor as soon as I could. He said I needed surgery to insert a miniature implant to replace the failing bone and put a tube in my ear for drainage.

I lay in bed feeling sorry for myself. How could I, a health professional who was always advising people on their health, be so unhealthy?

Then, the realization dawned. I had taken care of everyone else except myself.

Weeks later, I had the operation on the left ear, and everything improved. But the implant later failed after being pulled off the bone by scar tissue. Luckily, the highly skilled surgeon was able to find enough space to replace it and restore some hearing. I returned to work.

Later, I had the right ear done, and was delighted not only to hear better, but also not to have to wear a hearing aid again. This enabled me to work as a physiotherapist for a further twelve years.

Finally, I had my last hearing test. It was my surgeon's time to be surprised. He said the surgery had really improved my hearing. And I agreed it had, but added that I had also done a lot of work to calm myself and reduce my anxiety.

He confirmed that an overactive nervous system and brain can affect one's hearing. And I continued to meditate and work on breathing and relaxation techniques that helped loosen my neck, jaw, and shoulders. I also learned to slow down.

At the time, I was like a lot of busy mothers, trying to juggle family and career. My stress levels must have been through the roof, which was why my health was poor. And I wish I had realized that earlier and taken action sooner.

During all my health issues, I was reminded how traumatic incidents in one's life can impact long-term well-being. For example, while I was on a trail ride at school in England, a fellow rider fell off her horse, hit her head on the curb, and instantly died. I was devastated emotionally and had terrible survivor's guilt.

Later, my brother committed suicide while at university, just before I was taking my final physiotherapy exams. This was a tragic loss for me and my parents, leaving unanswered questions that linger to this day.

Then, I emigrated to Canada, which offered me a fresh start, but threw up its own hardships and challenges.

I decided to try an alternative approach to the one offered by conventional medicine, and found a highly trained craniosacral therapist who also happened to be a physiotherapist. Craniosacral therapy is a gentle, hands-on approach that releases tensions deep in the body to relieve pain and dysfunction. It's a manual technique pioneered by American osteopath John E. Upledger, and it has its critics. However, I have found it to be very helpful, at least as a starting point. It certainly improved the drainage for my eustachian tubes.

Those craniosacral therapy sessions proved to be one of the stepping stones towards my eventual independence from any further medical support for my ear conditions. But I believe it was the fact that I was now on a mission to help myself that really put me in the driver's seat.

Like other patients, I hated having to sit in one doctor's office after another, only to be told I was a "complicated" case. We are all complex people with sometimes complicated conditions. I just wanted to get straight to the root of the problem . . . by learning more about it myself.

I found what was helpful, too, was imagining a ball of healing energy circling around my head from one ear to the other. In fact, the more I treated my body as a whole, the less I thought about my ears.

In hindsight, I believe I could have done more for myself earlier on, rather than waiting for a crisis. On the other hand, my prolonged adversity has served me well in understanding the plight of others seeking help for their own health battles.

Serious health issues often start with an episode, trauma, or period of stress. Then, medications are prescribed, which may provide some relief, but often fail to solve the underlying issue.

My advice to you is to solve your own little riddles as you go.

Problems

- Putting all the power in the hands of the medical system.
- Inherited health issues.
- Recurring ear infections.
- Over-prescription of antibiotics.
- Gut and skin issues.

Solutions

- Taking more responsibility for my own health.
- Simplifying "complicated" cases.
- Tackling health problems early.
- Exploring alternative approaches.
- Treating the body as a whole.

CHAPTER 3

Beating the Odds with Cancer

The way some people deal with the sudden onset of a life-changing health condition is nothing short of inspirational. And one of my best friends has a lesson for us all in the way she took charge of her life after being diagnosed with brain cancer.

Her name is Jane Morgan, a retired realtor who lives in the wine-growing district of Kelowna in southern British Columbia. When she was sixty-three, she and her husband, Duncan, and their two dogs embarked on a six-month trip around the United States.

They bought a forty-foot motorhome, rented out their house, and set off on what should have been the adventure of a lifetime.

"We traveled south across the United States border into Washington State, staying overnight in a lovely forestry department campground. The following day, we drove into

Oregon where we met up with friends for several days, before heading to California," Jane said.

They stopped at an RV park in Buellton, California, for a couple of nights, and went to an Italian restaurant.

"After a lovely evening, we got back to the RV park and went to bed," she told me. "And two hours later, I apparently had a grand mal seizure."

Duncan called for an ambulance, and Jane woke up two hours later in hospital in Solvang, about twenty minutes away from Buellton. She did not realize where she was . . . and became frightened.

Luckily, the small village hospital had just received an MRI machine. So, she had a head scan, which revealed a small growth in her brain, and was transferred by ambulance to a hospital in Santa Barbara at 4:00 a.m.

"After several more scans and visits from four specialist doctors, I was told my best course of action would be to return home immediately, get my affairs in order, and consult with a neurosurgeon," she said.

The Santa Barbara medical staff did not reveal exactly what their diagnosis was, but Jane figured it would be cancer.

Duncan spoke to them privately, and they were apparently not that optimistic about a full recovery. Obviously, he kept this to himself before calling ahead to Jane's family doctor in Kelowna, who arranged for her to meet a surgeon as soon as possible.

The next day, Jane flew out of Los Angeles International Airport on her own. And the following day, armed with the MRI results from Santa Barbara, she went to the Kelowna surgeon. He told her she did indeed have cancer, consisting of a small stage-two tumour. And he immediately booked her in for surgery.

"I felt very calm about the whole thing," she said. "I knew I would survive; I felt it at a cellular level. I believed this was another lesson I had to learn. I've had many lessons to learn over the years, coping with several different stressful situations and having had an unhappy childhood."

The surgery went well, and Jane felt well. She underwent radiation and chemotherapy for a couple of years. She tried to resist taking this. But as her family, her doctor, and her specialists all told her, it was the only treatment available. And the cancer would probably return if she didn't take it.

The hospital had brain-cancer-survivor classes, which she could have attended, but chose not to, because she imagined it would make her believe she still had cancer.

"I lived as though I had never had cancer. I never acknowledged it. It had just 'visited,' " she said. "My life changed. I was unable to drive for two years after the seizure, so Duncan had to take me everywhere, even to get a coffee."

For someone who was a busy, independently minded person, this was tough to accept. But she got through it.

"I just stayed very positive and had no pain to cope with, which obviously helped," she said. "I never worried about being sick or having any side-effects. As far as I was concerned, I was fit and healthy. My total focus was on being well. Instead of 'waging war' on the cancer, I accepted it as having been part of my body, and just got on with living my life."

She joined an online group called Cure for Cancer, which helped her become more informed. And she reverted to vegetarianism.

She gave up alcohol, kept to an alkaline diet regime, avoided sugar whenever possible, and bought mostly local and organic foods. She began taking supplements such as omega-3 fatty acids.

"I carried on exercising, playing tennis, walking several miles every day, and painting," she said. "It's been seven years since this happened and I'm in remission; it seems like a distant memory, though I will be taking anti-seizure medication for the rest of my life, and my semi-annual (soon to be annual) MRI is a reminder of my journey."

Jane credits her recovery to the superb medical care she received both in Canada and the United States, which she says has "a brilliant system if you can afford it."

Her medical insurance covered the entire cost of $35,000 US for the two days she spent in hospital in the United States, plus the two ambulance trips she took.

"My Canadian neurosurgeon is one of the best in Canada, and luckily for me he lives in Kelowna," she said. "The

Kelowna General Hospital oncologists were highly professional and very caring."

She added, "I think the combination of excellent medical care, my strength of character, and refusal to accept that I would be unwell brought me through . . . together with a few changes in lifestyle. So far, all is well, and I'm sure it always will be."

Jane's story is a great example of taking the best of what both the American and Canadian medical systems have to offer and following their recommendations.

But it doesn't stop there. She made her own decisions about her health, changed her diet, kept active, and remained highly disciplined in all aspects of her long-term recovery.

Overall, though, I think perhaps her greatest asset was her iron will and fierce determination to prevail. Her courage shines through.

Problems

○ Sudden life-shattering event.

○ Fear of the unknown.

○ Juggling two medical systems.

○ Loss of independence.

○ Coping with cancer.

Solutions

○ Keeping calm and believing in yourself.

○ Seeking the best medical help.

○ Charting your own recovery course.

○ Considering changing your diet.

○ Not overlooking the power of exercise

CHAPTER 4

Determination through
Knee Pain

During the course of my long physiotherapy career, I have learned that tenacity and the desire to get well often help patients overcome apparently overwhelming obstacles.

Cynthia, a British Columba teacher, acknowledged that she was a somewhat sedentary person. Tired after a day in the classroom, she preferred reading and chatting to friends rather than working out or staying active in other ways.

As a result, she was losing a lot of lower-body strength and starting to complain about pain in both her knees. In fact, she was becoming so weak she worried she might not be able to get around without a walker.

Little things like standing up, going up and down stairs, and getting up off the toilet were becoming difficult for her. It was little wonder she was frustrated.

Cynthia told me her doctor had prescribed anti-inflammatory medications, but they were not really helping. And several of her friends were saying she should think about having knee-replacement surgery.

Whoa!

I suggested first doing a thorough physical assessment, from top to toe, to find out what was going on. She agreed this would be better than scurrying off to have a disruptive operation.

My assessment revealed that Cynthia had some arthritis in her knees. But it was the lack of strength in her legs, hips, core, and upper back that was leaving her joints unsupported and irritated.

I did some hands-on treatment, gave her a set of exercises for her joint stiffness, and suggested some elastic-band routines she could do every day at home.

I explained that she also needed to tune up her balance mechanism, and showed her how to supple and strengthen her feet and ankles . . . and restore her arches. I also told her how to realign her body and restore her gait as she became increasingly sure-footed.

For the first month, Cynthia saw little reduction in her pain and no apparent improvement in her overall stability. "I'm about to give up on this," she told me.

However, I replied, "You've done the hard part, which was getting started and committing to a consistent regimen. And now you just have to stay the course, and I know you will come through this."

Eight weeks later, she came into the physiotherapy clinic, beaming. "Thank you," she said. "Finally, I can feel the difference. I know I am getting stronger and can do quite a bit more, and my pain is decidedly less."

The fact is she was all but cured. No surgery was needed. And the person she had most to thank for this was herself.

I have spent four decades working as a physiotherapist. And my main conclusion about patients' outcomes is that those who accept professional guidance and take responsibility for their own health recover the quickest and best.

They are the people like Cynthia who are prepared to do the consistent, hard work that it takes to succeed in bringing their body back into balance.

I advised Cynthia to continue with her exercises until she could do nearly everything she wanted. I stressed that she should do the prescribed exercises regularly to keep her muscles in tune.

Many patients, though, are simply looking for a quick fix. And once they feel better, they tend to stop doing the treatment routine that's helped them. They then become slaves to their old habits and patterns of movement . . . and their pain returns.

Sadly, they soon find themselves well on the way to becoming the *forever patients* that I mentioned earlier.

My intention in writing this book is not to embarrass or harshly criticize anyone. Which is why, in several instances, I have been careful to guard patients' privacy by changing their names and altering personal details that might serve to identify them.

I simply wish to use my medical experience to pass on a few key suggestions that should enable you to improve your body awareness and overall well-being.

The health-care system, though life-saving at times, can end up making you dependent on medications and surgical operations that could be avoided if your condition were managed better from the get-go.

Pharmaceutical pills can certainly help patients recover from an acute, painful episode. But generally they do not provide long-term solutions.

In fact, those over-the-counter or prescription anti-inflammatory medications some people pop like candy may do serious damage to their liver and kidneys.

A cautionary note here: I certainly do not want you to be reckless with your health. If you are in pain and are concerned about it, you should seek swift medical attention.

However, I would strongly suggest you learn as much as possible about your body and how it functions best. This will prove invaluable in managing the ups and downs we all go through.

As for surgery, by all means use the incredible procedures we now have available to us. But do not submit to the surgeon's knife to relieve joint pains and back issues before you have tried non-invasive treatments given by physio-therapists or other highly trained professionals. Tackle these issues sooner rather than later.

During her last treatment, Cynthia told me she had not realized how committed she had to be to stick with the regime I recommended. She admitted she was about to give up on it, because she felt it wasn't working.

She only took her recovery seriously when I explained there is no such thing as an instant cure for a long-term problem, and that it would take several weeks of exercises for her to regain the strength she needed.

She stuck with the program, became pain-free, and earned a new lease on life.

Problems

○ Sedentary lifestyle.

○ Lack of strength and balance.

○ Believing there's a quick fix.

○ Being overdependent on medications.

Solutions

○ Making a firm health commitment.

○ Learning more about your body.

○ Having a plan and sticking with it.

○ Working hard for change.

CHAPTER 5

Taking Control of Neck Stiffness and Dizziness

Patrick was a quiet, respectful, middle-aged man referred to me by another therapist. Outwardly he looked fine, but he said he was increasingly bothered by headaches and the overall state of his health.

He explained he suffered from dizziness, which is among the most common reasons people see their doctor. There are many causes of dizziness, making it important to get a diagnosis. He also had occasional bouts of vertigo (where he felt he or his surroundings were spinning). His balance was poor, and his neck was stiff and sore on one side. His shoulders were very tight.

Patrick added that he did a lot of driving for his job, and suffered from stress. "I'm just really scared with what's going on in my life," he told me. "I don't know how I'm going to fix this." He did seem genuinely scared.

After doing an overall balance assessment, I asked him if he'd ever had a neck injury. He said he had, when he was much younger.

I treated him with manual traction, soft-tissue and postural realignment techniques, and gave him exercises to restore his equilibrium.

He told me he found the physio treatments helpful. But I warned him that he was caught in a quandary in that his dizziness made him anxious—and his anxiety made him dizzy and tense. Then, he tended to panic.

I recommended that, when he suffered one of these attacks, he should attempt to relax and breathe slowly from his belly. I said this might seem counterintuitive, but it would help calm the flight-fight area of his brain, the amygdala.

He tried the relaxed breathing I suggested, and it really seemed to work. Then, I discussed with him how his stressful job was likely worsening his condition, which could get even worse unless he decided to tackle it. And that would not be easy, I said, because he would have to put in extra effort to alter the way he approached life. I asked him to decide what he thought would be the best plan for himself.

Patrick's eyes lit up. He seemed to appreciate fully that there was a way out of this, if he was willing to take it.

First, he said he wanted to talk to his doctor about reducing the dosage of the drugs he had been prescribed, to make him less dependent on them. Then, he started doing the exercises I recommended and began to take steps to reduce his overall stress.

Patrick's case reminded me that, to deal with complex health problems, patients need a correct diagnosis from an attentive doctor or other medical professional able to recommend a treatment regimen.

Patient engagement and empowerment are key. And my view is that those who accept the reality of their condition and are prepared to take ownership of it are twice as likely to recover as those who are looking for a quick fix.

The next time I saw Patrick he was not only doing well, but working for himself. He had started his own business, and was happy doing so, even though it was all new to him. He felt more in control of his life.

Though he was never keen on doing formal exercises, he took his dog for daily walks and was doing exercises to help his balance as well as eye and head movements, posture and relaxation. His dizziness had improved significantly and so had his work-life balance.

Later, he would come and see me occasionally to stretch his neck and release his tight muscles. And it was wonderful to see him go from being a very worried man to someone who was happy, healthy and at peace with himself.

Problems

○ Dizziness, occasional vertigo, headaches, and neck pain.

○ Stress, anxiety, and poor sleep.

○ Stressful job involving too much driving.

○ Too many medications.

○ Feeling a loss of control.

Solutions

○ Reviewing medications with the doctor.

○ Taking physio treatments, including vestibular rehabilitation.

○ Reducing stress.

○ Controlling anger.

○ Switching careers.

○ Ongoing monitoring by a family doctor.

○ Changing lifestyle.

CHAPTER 6

A Holistic Approach to a Healthy Pelvic Floor and Sex Life

My experience is that people seriously underestimate the link between mental stress and physical discomfort. This is clearly evident with the pelvic floor, which governs the body's major functions.

Television bombards us with advertising for the pads that supposedly solve the common problem of "bladder leakage."

But these pads treat only the symptoms of the condition—not its root causes—and lead women to think there are no other options, except possibly surgery.

The fact is, though, that stress incontinence can be treated successfully, especially if patients—both men and women—seek out a professional who specializes in pelvic-floor health and offers a holistic solution addressing its physical and emotional aspects.

Anniken Chadwick is a women's health physiotherapist who lives and works in British Columbia, and specializes in this area. Here's what she told me.

> *The pelvic floor is the most emotionally charged and misunderstood muscle group in the body—misunderstood because it is often treated like an all-or-nothing muscle that should be on and strong at all times, which is not the case.*
>
> *It's emotionally charged because it is wired that way as part of our anxiety-stress-fear response. If you are watching a scary movie and all your muscles were hooked up to an electromyography (EMG) machine, they would tense as you anticipated the threat. But your pelvic floor would tense much more so than the rest of your muscles.*
>
> *Think of the pelvic floor as your tail-wagger. Any experience or activity where your tail would go between your legs causes pelvic tensing. This could be anything from minor stresses to major trauma, from being late for work to sexual abuse.*
>
> *All muscles develop patterns. So, if you are tensing because of current life stresses or past trauma, they can get stuck in a state of permanent tension. If your pelvic floor is stuck in tension, it can't work well.*
>
> *Take a common patient scenario I see: Client A, let's call her Angela, comes in two years after giving birth.*

She has stress incontinence and is frustrated as she's done many pelvic-floor exercises, but they're not helping. She also has painful sex, so she avoids it as much as possible, and her libido has decreased considerably.

On assessment, Angela's pelvic floor is really tight. A tight muscle can't contract any further, so when she runs and needs the contraction of the floor to support her bladder, there's no power left. And the bladder leaks from the impact of the bounce. Furthermore, to try and stop herself from leaking, she tenses everything and this prevents the natural movement of her trunk and hips.

The tension creates more pressure onto her bladder, and actually causes Angela to leak more. So, the more she tries to stop leaking, the more she pushes pee out of her bladder. At the same time, the way she is holding her body is inhibiting the pelvic floor. So, of course, the leaking just gets worse.

So why might her pelvic floor be tense in the first place? It's fairly normal to have a tense pelvic floor after the straining involved in giving birth.

For C-sections, the lower-abdomen scar can also cause the floor to protectively tighten.

After giving birth, Angela didn't realize she was tight and that her Kegel exercises [named after US gynecologist Arnold Kegel] were making her tighter. When she tried penetrative sex for the first time with her husband, the tightness made her sore and caused her pelvic floor to tighten up even more to protect itself.

This made it still sorer, and the vicious cycle got worse. In the end, her whole pelvic floor was tensing at the thought of having sex, in anticipation of the pain.

Along with the tensing to stop leaking and all the Kegels, the anticipation of pain—and likely some post-partum stress—had created continual tension down there. Her pelvic floor was tight, sensitive, and over-reactive, and its natural functioning was thrown off completely.

What does Angela need to do? Well, she needs to let go of the constant tensing, even though she's afraid that might make her leak more.

In the physio clinic, we assessed her pelvic floor, and I was able to release some of the tension. This greatly improved her strength, because she could do a big contraction from a relaxed state.

She continued to work on her exercises, but with a focus on teaching her brain how to relax the pelvic-floor muscles. In doing this, she eventually started to notice when she was tight, which helped reduce her chronic tensing habit.

We also looked at her posture and running mechanics, and found she had tightness through her chest and upper back. This was creating excess downward pressure on the bladder, increasing the chance of leaking. To run, you need to be able to twist your back. So, when we loosened this area, it improved her hip mechanics and took pressure off the bladder.

The pelvic floor can only work if the hips are in the right biomechanical position, so it's important to correct them in order to let the pelvic floor do its thing. Otherwise, it's like fixing a wonky window frame in a house where the foundation is totally off. You'd be fixing it forever and it would never be fully right.

Angela learned to let go of her pelvic floor, opened up her chest and upper back, and retrained her breath and running gait, all of which took the pressure off her bladder. This also allowed her pelvic floor to engage appropriately and she stopped leaking when running.

Now for the sex part. Sometimes the pelvic floor can have a long memory when it comes to pain and/or trauma. Once that anticipatory protective response is built in, it can take a lot of mindfulness to override it.

We worked on rebuilding her pleasure pathways. That meant engaging in sexual activity with her husband that didn't involve any penetration, to decrease the fear of association.

The relaxing pelvic-floor muscle exercises really helped with Angela's awareness of when she was tightening. But if they had continued just trying for penetrative sex, she would still feel it tightening involuntarily, and this would have made sex more painful.

We worked with vaginal dilators so she could practise putting something in her vagina (very small and narrow at first, then slowly increasing the girth) while staying safe and relaxed in her body.

Over time, she gained confidence and skill in being able to stop the pre-emptive tensing. This helped reduce her fear avoidance around sex and increased her libido, too.

Angela was able to get up to a dilator the same girth as her husband's penis when he was erect. And as her desire returned, she worked with her husband to have pleasurable, penetrative sex again.

Many other women experience the same problems or a variation thereof, but suffer in silence. What's also fairly common is that these issues are fixable.

It is estimated that one in three women have stress urinary incontinence at some time in their lives.

Angela's successful treatment, outlined above by Anniken, highlights the need for people to avoid quick, superficial fixes and to educate themselves fully about their condition.

The combination of self-help and professional help seems to work best.

Problems

○ Embarrassment and loss of libido.

○ Patients' misconceptions about Kegel exercises.

○ Delays in seeing a professional specializing in the pelvic floor.

○ The emotional aspect of stress incontinence.

○ Painful penetrative sex with her husband.

Solutions

○ Making an appointment with a women's health professional skilled in this area.

○ Getting an assessment and making a follow-up plan.

○ Reprogramming pelvic floor muscles.

○ Increasing libido with relaxation and stretching exercises.

○ Making sure the treatment plan achieves its goal.

Curiosity Works even with Severe Stomach Pain

Sophie was a patient of mine. She was an energetic, elegant, and fun-loving woman who had recently retired from a demanding job for a large corporation. She looked forward to going to the gym, hiking, and enjoying life with her friends and family.

She always liked making a difference in people's lives, and did her fair share of volunteering. However, she started to have stomach problems that were so serious she could not eat anything without pain.

She went to her family doctor, who diagnosed her with acid reflux and gave her various medications, none of which, she said, made any difference.

Then, she was referred to a gastroenterologist. But still her stomach acted up badly, and she found it hard to eat anything at all without great discomfort.

"I started hating cooking and realized my relationship with food was beginning to affect me psychologically. I'd watch people eat food I used to love, and I would cry. Many times, I would call my mom and have a good cry as it seemed there wasn't anyone willing to help me," she told me.

Finally, Sophie decided to take charge of her own health and found a new family doctor. This doctor listened to her and referred her to a new gastroenterologist. This time, she received a diagnosis that was the opposite of the first. She was told the sphincter to her stomach had gone into spasm and would not open to receive the food.

She was given the option of Botox injections or surgery. She opted for the former, and received some relief, finding she was able to eat more normally. She also went on her own recovery journey, doing what her new specialist doctor recommended, namely to reconnect her brain to her eating.

I asked Sophie when the problem with her stomach started. She said it was when she was away in Montreal with her family and was feeling anxious about her coming retirement.

Her condition had involved her vagus nerve, the largest cranial nerve in the body. It signals to the brain and gut that it's safe to rest and digest or, conversely, to flee. The nerve, it seemed, was being triggered by all her anxiety. Sophie needed to learn to switch on the rest-and-digest response (parasympathetic nervous system) and switch off the fight-or-flight one (sympathetic nervous system).

Sophie learned to do this nerve-calming manoeuvre through diaphragmatic breathing exercises, meditation, and mindful eating. She no longer watched the TV news at mealtimes or did anything to interfere with eating being a pleasurable experience. Sophie found these links helpful to her: mayoclinic.org and badgut.org. Also see Weight, Diet, and Digestion in chapter 14.

When she told me her story, I agreed that these relaxation exercises were exactly what she needed to do. I simply reinforced her belief in her self-help journey. She was soon able to overcome her debilitating stomach problem and felt comforted in the knowledge that, in fact, she would not need surgery.

Sophie said she found some useful information online, and that the combination of sound medical guidance and her own curiosity worked very well. Also, taking the initiative to go on a discovery mission made her feel more powerful and in control of her life. This helped her immeasurably.

"A lot of research spoke to proper eating habits—not eating in a hurry, but chewing properly and staying away from distractions like TV, iPhones, and computers while eating," she explained. "I found an article connecting the vagus nerve and the part it plays in proper digestion. As I did more research, I began to examine my eating habits and realized I had some particularly bad ones."

She realized her emotional state had a major impact on her digestive process. Instead of standing up and wolfing down her food, she now consciously sits down to eat.

"I relax and take time to be aware of eating, chewing, and tasting my food; and I don't rush when I am finished," she said. "I realized I was constantly under stress and never took time to let my digestive system do its job."

The suggestion by Sophie's second gastroenterologist that she practise diaphragmatic breathing to relax her digestive system and her mind proved a game-changer. While it took her time to see its benefits, this type of breathing is now her go-to exercise for any tummy trouble or anxiety.

Sophie added she is cautious when researching online websites: "Many of them contradict each other and are poorly written. I found the Mayo clinic website to be an excellent resource."

Fortunately, she added, one of her good friends is a retired medical professional to whom she could refer her findings for validation.

"It has been a long, hard journey to this point," she said. "Taking control of my health by being assertive and not accepting advice from doctors who don't care to help has been my saving grace. The online research I did was very helpful."

Sophie's story illustrates how too many people eat their meals in a hurried, unsettled way, which is detrimental to their health. Sometimes, the way we eat can be as bad as what we eat.

So, are you taking your time to chew slowly? Well, digestion begins in the mouth, so consciously calm yourself down while you eat and don't scarf down your food on the run.

Above all, teach your children to sit and eat slowly with no distractions. Warm, loving, social, and relaxed eating is the best. A healthy diet is a bonus.

Problems

○ Fast, hurried eating resulting in stomach pain.

○ Stress, anxiety.

○ Unreliable online information.

○ Unsympathetic medical professional.

Solutions

○ Finding a good doctor.

○ Getting a correct diagnosis.

○ Learning more about yourself.

○ Refusing to accept personal limitations.

○ Learning to breathe, meditate, and relax.

CHAPTER 8

Reassurance Needed for
Back Pain

The first time I met this retired lawyer, George, I knew he was going to be a challenge. I could tell he wasn't going to suffer fools gladly. He asked me a series of questions about my credentials and experience.

Now in his seventies, he complained constantly of the back pain he had suffered for many years. He told me he was not an active man, but rather one who enjoyed classical music, reading books and newspapers, and having many opinions on many things.

The lawyer could be charming, but was testy. He hated more than anything to be told how well he looked, because he said he always felt unwell. My challenge was to listen to him and help him gently stretch his stiff back and legs. Also, I had to encourage him to breathe properly, go for daily walks, and generally become more active.

"You look well," he would say. "Well, actually I feel tired," I'd reply, mirroring his pessimism. And he would just laugh and smile.

I managed to persuade him to undertake a daily regimen of exercises and balance training to improve his stability, but he did so grudgingly. And he would become anxious and despondent when he was about to leave for his cabin or had to fly somewhere.

He would always return in one piece from these trips, and I would routinely ask how it went, to which he would always reply that, yes, it had all gone well, followed by a wry smile.

My job became to "reassure" him that his back was not going to seize up and become painful, and that he was going to be perfectly fine. I was not being reckless here. With all the testing and functional movements he was able to do, his main issue was his self-limiting belief.

George would see me intermittently, and mostly when he needed a dose of motivation or reassurance. His biggest fear was that he would end up in a wheelchair. Normally, joshing with a patient about this would not be funny. But for him, it deflated the elephant in the room, namely his fear of not being in control of his life anymore.

He carried on living remarkably well for a further ten years, until he started to develop dementia and had to go into a nursing home.

Mark Twain is quoted as saying, "I've had a lot of worries in my life, most of which never happened." And I was truly sorry the lawyer had spent so many years being fearful of his back condition and the impending doom he had concocted in his mind. If he'd been able to overcome his constant worries, he would have made life so much easier for himself and his wife.

Many other people, it's clear, also have this kind of fear. The lawyer, in fact, reminds me of my father-in-law, a professional musician whom I first met when I was a physiotherapy student at London's Middlesex Hospital.

He used to sit a lot at the piano, and then would ask me about his bad back. I gave him detailed instructions and suggested exercises he could do to ease his pain and stiffness. And every time I would visit, he would bring out a pristine piece of paper with my list of exercises. But he never did any of them!

The fact is if you live a sedentary lifestyle and don't exercise much, there's a good chance you will become stiff and sore in your spine, hips, or elsewhere in your body. Your general balance will suffer, and you won't want to move. This inactivity brings with it a host of unwanted chronic conditions that could be avoided with walking and movement.

Besides, if you find you're gradually allowing your body to succumb to the forces of gravity, the chances are you'll adopt what's known as the "walker posture." And someone will suggest you should walk using one of those metal walking frames that old or ill people use to help them walk.

To check this, look at your reflection in a shop window while you are passing by. If you notice you are stooping, try bringing yourself more upright. This will encourage your buttocks, legs, abdominals, and upper back to become strong enough to resist the forces of gravity. But the longer you wait to do this, the harder it gets. Unfortunately, until you see how you are standing, sitting, and generally moving, your brain will believe you are upright when you are not. When you see the faulty movements and postures, this will give your brain important visual feedback. Training and repetition will help you develop self-awareness and conscious movement. See the balance and posture exercises in my book, *The Posture Pain Fix*.

The body relies on steady, regular movement to lubricate its joints, move oxygen from the heart and lungs to the rest of the body and provide nutrition to all its cells, while removing toxins and other waste via the kidneys, liver, and lymphatic system. Exercise is definitely the best medicine, especially when coupled with regular reassurance and positive reinforcement.

One of my more anxious patients was Victoria, a teacher who was worried about recurring pain and having a fragile back. She was a highly intelligent, sensitive woman who had been plagued by lower-back pain ever since her son was born—he was now an older teenager.

I saw her as a patient for a while before I was able to show and convince her, through the right movement patterns, that she had more control over her back than she thought. Earlier, several other health professionals had told her that her pelvis was unstable and that her back was weak. And, naturally, she believed them.

Victoria did, in fact, have poor muscle control around her back, hips, and legs. However, fear of moving an "unstable" pelvis was the picture she created in her mind, which convinced her that her spine would collapse with any wrong movement.

Her son was moving away to university in the United States, and she planned to drive him there to help settle him in. Her back, of course, started to act up, because of all her worry over her boy leaving home for the first time. She felt overwhelmed, and was in tears wondering how she was going to manage it all.

Just before she left, I spent time familiarizing her with different positions that didn't cause her any pain. I showed her how to move her hips, knees, and ankles, and how to keep her spine stacked up in a balanced way.

She was learning what we physiotherapists call "correct body mechanics." And she seemed reassured.

I advised Victoria to use any pain she did suffer as her guide, or at least a reminder, that she wasn't moving in the right way. The next day, she drove her son to his university, a day-and-a-half's journey.

I saw her on her return and she was beaming. Her journey had gone well. She had broken the trip up into one-hour chunks so she could regularly get out of the car and move around. Her son was happy, and she felt heartened that her back was tougher than she had thought. It was a life-changing confidence booster.

The moral of this story is to trust yourself and help others trust in themselves. In my experience, patients gain a huge amount of confidence from the realization that their body comes alive when they begin to move it correctly. Then, their pain starts to subside and they feel younger and more in control.

Problems

○ Allowing a diagnosis or assessment to remain permanently when it no longer serves you.

○ Being overly fearful of spine damage or severe pain.

○ Becoming fixated on a single health issue.

○ Not being willing to try a different approach.

Solutions

○ Remaining hopeful and optimistic.

○ Finding skilled professionals who will give you the confidence to recover.

○ Believing you will regain your health.

CHAPTER 9

Feeling Trapped by Chronic Shoulder Pain

Pamela, a home-based computer worker, was under a great deal of stress when her husband developed a terminal disease. Before he died, she drove him to various medical appointments and had to help him get in and out of bed. Now, she herself was starting to suffer from chronic shoulder pain.

During this tough time, she experienced increasing health, financial and work pressures. She was stuck between a rock and a hard place.

Also, she had two aging parents to take care of, though they lived in their own home. Her stubborn father refused outside help for himself or his wife. And she had a married son with struggles of his own. She was run off her feet.

I saw Pamela weekly, and the physiotherapy I gave her was keeping her shoulder from freezing. But it wasn't helping her overcome her debilitating pain or the difficulty she was having getting a good night's sleep.

Her family doctor prescribed pain and anti-inflammatory medications, which also were not helping much.

A different approach was clearly needed. I suggested to Pamela that she needed to take steps to reduce her stress level—and that, if she didn't, she was heading for major health problems. Already, she had been diagnosed as a borderline diabetic, no doubt because of her sedentary, stressed lifestyle.

I suggested she take a good look at her life and decide for herself what steps would unburden her heavy load and allow her to feel in charge. She later concluded, after much thought, that the best option for her was to de-clutter the house and sell it before moving into a nearby apartment.

She also quit her job, because she now had the money from the home sale to enable her to retire. This lifted a load off her shoulders, and her overall health started to dramatically improve.

I've treated scores of patients who are dealing with exceedingly trying circumstances; many of them fill me with admiration for the way they do so. Pamela did more than just cope. She made a herculean effort to regain her good health.

She succeeded in what she was determined to do. And I applaud her for it.

Her story highlights the way our health tends to mirror our lifestyle, for better or for worse. Sedentary people who are feeling blocked at work will often experience back pain.

Constant financial struggles can lead to problems ranging from knotted muscles to stiff necks and sleeplessness. And domestic issues, including raising challenging teenagers, can literally give one headaches.

"I felt completely trapped and could see no end to my stress; my health was suffering. I decided if I didn't change my situation voluntarily, circumstances would change it for me," Pamela said. "I now feel so much better and in charge of my life again."

Increasingly, health professionals are speaking out about the link between health and lifestyle.

Dr. Monique Tello, a Harvard Medical School clinical instructor, says improving your diet, managing stress, increasing activity, and sleeping well can lead to better, longer lives. Eating a plant-based diet, for example, can lower inflammation.

"Simply put, food is medicine," Tello notes in the Harvard Health Blog. "Some doctors are providing this information to patients as part of their regular medical care."

So, if you find you are not recovering from the pain or other condition you are being treated for, ask yourself whether you are under duress, stress, or might have a lot of inflammation in your system. Under these circumstances, your body will likely not recover the way it should.

Problems

○ Family and work stress.

○ Loss of a loved one.

○ Money problems.

○ Feeling lonely and trapped.

○ Parents, children and grandchildren needing support.

○ A cluttered home.

○ Lack of exercise.

Solutions

○ Decluttering.

○ Financial restructuring.

○ Selling the family home and purchasing a condo.

○ Giving up a stressful job.

○ Exercising and making other lifestyle changes.

○ Making time for family and friends.

CHAPTER 10

Conscious Breathing to Control Pain

B reathing is something we really can't live without. We live hurried, breathless lives, but filling our lungs with air is as essential to living as singing is to an opera. We take around 25,000 breaths a day.

Have you ever wondered why women used to die from pneumonia? Well, in the pursuit of beauty, they wore corsets that strangled their rib cages. And when they got chest infections, they were unable to breathe deeply and effectively enough to remove mucous from their lungs and cough it out. Sadly, this would often lead to their death.

With the COVID-19 pandemic and all the variants that will continue to evolve, our breathing needs to be kept in tip-top condition more than ever.

Fear only makes us take quick, short, shallow breaths. Instead, we should be learning to use the whole of our lungs by inhaling air into our bellies and making full use of our diaphragm, the large dome-shaped muscle that separates the abdomen from the chest.

We need this muscle, the diaphragm, for inspiration, for breathing in. Expanding our rib cage presses down on our internal, abdominal organs to make room for the air to come into our lungs. That is why it is so important not to slump our back and compress our organs thereby inhibiting the diaphragm's ability to work.

Sitting and/or standing with an open, tall torso allows the belly to expand and lets oxygen enter our lungs, one important breath after another. And good breathing greatly helps in controlling pain, as charismatic, convention planner Lucy found to her relief.

I remember the day Lucy came to see me, because she had a bravado that masked her stress. In her mid-forties, she enjoyed her stressful occupation: "I rather like being on the edge of my seat and bringing everything together for the 'big weekend' when the conventions are held."

She told me that on one side of her rib cage she had developed a pain that was radiating into her upper back. It was bothering her day and night. Nighttime ribcage pain can be particularly uncomfortable because, in bed, the rib cage takes the weight of the torso when a person is lying on their side.

Lucy had a slight curvature in her spine, and her mid-back was very stiff. She found it hard to turn from her torso and look behind her, and her breathing pattern was poor.

She admitted that, while sitting at her computer, she constantly leaned to the same side, propping her head on her cupped hand and putting weight onto her elbow. It's a common habit that becomes more pronounced and more painful with repetition. And she realized she needed help.

By using my hands to gently relax Lucy's rib cage, I guided her to improve her breathing by encouraging her breathing muscles and rib joints to begin working again.

I also suggested she become more aware of her breathing patterns, to which she giggled, "Oh, I've never had to think about my breathing before."

I replied, "Unfortunately, we all tend to neglect doing the obvious thing. It's rather like when a machine is not working, we forget to check if it's plugged in!"

As journalist James Nestor points out in his book, *Breath: The New Science of a Lost Art*, the coronavirus has highlighted respiratory illnesses and the need to learn to breathe properly. He says "slow and low" breaths through the nose can help relieve stress and reduce blood pressure.

Nestor told National Public Radio that he himself took part in a study in which his nose was plugged for ten days, forcing him to breathe only through his mouth. "I developed sleep apnea," he said. "My stress levels were off the charts. My nervous system was a mess. I felt awful."

He added that a neuropsychologist had explained to him that anxious people typically breathe far too much: "So what happens when you breathe too much is you're constantly putting yourself into a state of stress."

Lucy acknowledged she needed to do more exercise to reduce her anxiety and make her stressful work life easier. "I'm too sedentary and too intense."

Fortunately, she said her pain diminished considerably after her first visit with me. But she still needed to remind herself constantly to become more breath-aware.

I suggested she notice how her body reacted to stress and to monitor how this affected her breathing. She also changed the way she tended to lean to one side.

The result was that she regained full health after three or four brief visits. And when I bumped into her on the street a few months later, she said she was feeling great and breathing productively.

Gerald, another patient of mine, was a middle-aged accountant who came into my clinic with acute lower back pain. He was literally breathless. He was so stiff and tense he could hardly move, and was obviously in great distress. In fact, I had to tell him gently that he was too wound up for me to examine him.

I explained to him that one of the best ways to reduce his pain was simply to breathe slowly and deeply from his belly and allow his tense muscles to relax and let go. Later, he admitted to me that this was a turning point in his recovery.

Being able to feel in charge of his pain, Gerald said, gave him a much-needed measure of control. "I wasn't as helpless as I thought," he said.

Remember shallow breathing promotes the fight or flight response whereas slow, deep, relaxed breathing helps with rest and digest and pain control.

Problems

- Slumping over a computer or other electronic device can restrict breathing.
- Poor breathing saps physical energy and drains mental capacity.
- Stress caused by bad breathing causes aches, pains, and other health problems.

Solutions

- Telling our heart and other vital organs to relax by belly breathing.
- Understanding how good breathing reduces stress and lowers blood pressure.
- Exercising to enhance deep breathing, which is one of the soundest health prescriptions.

CHAPTER 11

Hip Surgery Is No Quick Fix

The flip side to stories of health recovery and other successes are those of people who take the line of least resistance. Susan, a mother of two grown-up children, is one of those. She came to see me with a hip problem that was really bothering her.

She loved to take her dog for daily walks and play with her grandchildren. And she told me she couldn't deal anymore with the pain and disruption to her life that her painful limp and unnaturally tight muscles were causing her.

I examined her, and found she had the classic signs of an arthritic hip. Her sleep and daily activities were challenged. So, I discussed with her the lifestyle changes I thought she should make and gave her a specific, progressive balancing, strengthening, and stretching program to do regularly at home.

However, Susan would constantly recount stories to me about friends who took various medications to ease their pain, and how they knew people who had undergone surgery. Her friends told her not to bother with physiotherapy, as it was too much like hard work and wasn't going to solve her problem. It almost seemed as if getting a hip replacement in hospital was a badge of honour.

Unfortunately, she didn't appear to appreciate my contention that exercises, education, and balance work were going to help her. She tried the exercises a couple of times, felt they made little difference, and abandoned the protocol.

Despite my quoting recent evidence-based studies on the efficacy of exercises and education, Susan had her mind made up that surgery was her path to pain-free movement.

In this case, physiotherapy would prove to be a failure for Susan, who was clearly wanting a quick health fix. The last time I treated her she was already wait-listed for surgery. Later still, I heard she was having a second operation, this time for the other hip.

Like many patients, Susan seemed to believe that getting a hip replacement was child's play. But I can assure you that's far from the truth. Surgeries are by no means pain- or risk-free. And exercises are needed to get muscles strong again.

Hip replacements generally work out better than knee replacements, but sometimes tackling the pain and joint issues early with a well-researched method of rehabilitation is much better. Waiting until your hip is worn out and you can't stand it anymore is not the way to go.

Take Mary, for example, who at fifty-five started to have a lot of pain in her hip. She had difficulty walking, getting in and out of a chair, and standing up from the toilet. She was overweight, divorced, and had a son living away from home.

Mary had so much going for her, but I could tell she had some emotional issues . . . and that food gave her the comfort she seemed to crave.

She went to see one orthopaedic surgeon who told her she was too young to have a total hip replacement and she should tackle her weight and emotional issues first.

Mary decided to seek out a second opinion, and this second surgeon told her she should, indeed, have a total hip replacement.

He said that her new hip would last between ten and fifteen years, and that then she could return for a second hip replacement.

I think Mary liked this doctor's advice because it meant she could avoid tackling her personal issues and having to work to get her body strong again.

She did not understand that being overweight put her at risk for diabetes, heart ailments, and other medical problems.

My experience tells me that health issues often stem from emotional and lifestyle ones, and that the best ways to address both are to take stock of your life and regain control of your entire mental and physical well-being.

Surgery can be a lifesaver, but it's not something you should be relying on for regular, healthy, daily living.

Mary's son was urging her to have the surgery because he did not want to see his mother in pain. But neither did he like to see his mother overeating.

So what happens if the surgery is done, but the lifestyle issues are not addressed? All you will likely get is short-term relief, because the same underlying issues will remain. And you can't keep replacing every part of your body.

Some might argue that having an operation would allow you to move freely without pain, and, therefore, improve your overall health. That may be true for some patients, but my experience is it isn't generally the case.

The beauty of the human body is that, if you treat it right, it will mostly heal itself.

Don't take your body for granted. Learn as much as possible about the choices you have in taking care of it yourself . . . without surgical intervention, if possible.

Problems

○ Hip pain.

○ Sedentary lifestyle

○ Being overweight.

○ Lack of mobility.

○ Trying for a quick fix for long-term problems.

○ Looking to your non-expert friends for health advice.

○ Failing to consider evidence-based alternatives to surgery.

Solutions

○ Understanding the link between physical and mental pain.

○ Appreciating how chronic health problems often stem from lifestyle choices.

○ Being willing to seek out a variety of professional help.

CHAPTER 12

Gaming the System with Fraud

Most physiotherapists will tell you the most frustrating people to treat are those who don't seem to want to get better. Often, these patients have been in car crashes and are looking for an insurance settlement or extended time off work. So they feel they have to inflate the extent of their injuries.

Their lawyers emphasize what they cannot do, while their physiotherapist emphasizes what they can. So, there is a clash of expected outcomes, and sometimes the first casualty is the truth.

Now, I am not suggesting that legitimate injuries should not be compensated fairly. But I am pointing out that our Canadian, taxpayer-funded medical system has an ongoing problem with questionable claims, and more needs to be done to clamp down on this.

One patient referred to me was a young man who had been involved in what was described as a minor traffic accident. Tom worked as a carpet-layer, and he arrived at my clinic in apparent agony. I was unable to figure out what was causing him so much pain. Either he had an incredibly low pain threshold or he was magnifying his condition to show me how much he was suffering. Getting onto the treatment bed caused him to groan and wince. But, given the over-the-top nature of his reaction to my assessment, it was hard for me to pinpoint the cause of his pain. So, I gave him some advice about managing his soft-tissue injuries, and said I would contact his doctor.

A couple of days later, I happened to be driving along my neighbourhood parkway when I witnessed a man running athletically across the road. My mouth dropped as I turned my head to confirm that this was, indeed, Tom, the same man who could hardly get onto the treatment bed. Was this a miraculous recovery or was my hunch confirmed?

Tom never returned to the clinic to let me know. But clearly, the rising costs of treating soft-tissue injuries have been of concern to the British Columbia government. It recently introduced a $5,500 limit on payouts for pain and suffering following minor crashes to customers of the government-owned Insurance Corporation of British Columbia (ICBC).

Unfortunately, there are always those who think they can game the system—people like the middle-aged man,

Eustace, who came for a physio appointment because he, too, had been in a fairly minor car accident.

Now, I am not ignoring the fact that some supposedly minor soft-tissue injuries can cause more damage than is immediately obvious. But this patient was clearly exaggerating his condition as he walked into our clinic's curtained cubicle and seemed unable to move his upper body freely.

I asked him if he would like to proceed with the examination, explaining that, if he did, I would need him to take off his shirt and hang it on the peg above his chair. He agreed and, in doing so, managed to move his neck, shoulder, and arm with apparent ease. So, at least one problem was solved!

However, it is frustrating to try to help someone who is obviously more interested in obtaining compensation for their alleged injuries than in having them treated and improving their physical health. It's the kind of deception that can prove costly to taxpayers and is not fair to those who genuinely need medical help.

Still, I did give Eustace some of my professional advice. I also pointed out to him that I would be talking to his doctor about my observing him moving quite normally—which he proceeded to do even as he was leaving and returning to his car.

ICBC, meanwhile, notes that, whether by embellishing the extent of an injury or misrepresenting a previous medical condition, exaggerating a claim is a fraud.

"Most claims are honest," its website says, "but North American auto insurance industry studies estimate that 10 to 20 per cent of claims contain an element of fraud or exaggeration. This means that fraud is costing over $100 on every auto insurance policy."

Problems

○ People who don't want to get better.

○ Patients who exaggerate their injuries.

○ Patients only interested in compensation.

Solutions

○ Combatting rising taxpayer costs.

○ Raising public awareness.

CHAPTER 13

Stepping Up Your Health

Your health is a reflection of you. You are what you put in your body and how you cope with mental and physical issues. No one is going to care for you as well as you.

You cannot always rely on others to fix your underlying conditions. It's up to you to seek out the very best help, realizing that preventing problems is the key to addressing them. Fixing your body after it is broken is twice as hard as averting the injury or problem in the first place.

Humans are meant to move. You must avoid being sedentary. Sitting in front of a computer or TV for a long time will slowly ruin your health. You must do physical activities throughout your day. Your body needs regular movements to oxygenate, lubricate, and detoxify it.

Doctors and other health professionals are invaluable. But they won't necessarily be able to solve chronic health issues, as they can't fix everything (something they don't often like to admit). Also, they generally don't have the necessary training in those lifestyle issues that can greatly affect your health and well-being.

Taking the initiative to improve your own health will itself help make you better, no matter your age. If you have complex problems and are given the go-ahead by your doctor to work on your health, start with a small, achievable step. Your mind and body will react positively to the fact that you are finally taking control.

There is rarely such a thing as a quick fix to long-term health problems and the debilitating thought processes that often go with them. One way to overcome such challenges is through regular meditation. Another is to study various mind-body techniques.

I cannot emphasize enough that we need to become a mobile society, not a mobile-phone society. Stress and anxiety are becoming the norm for most people. People are living longer, but not necessarily better. But you can do a huge amount to improve the quality of your life, if you only know how.

You also need to be committed to do your part in following the recommendations you're given. And if they are not helping or are actually aggravating your condition, talk to your physiotherapist or other professional about your lack of progress. Don't just walk away. Instead, have the physio adjust your regimen. Just being given a sheet of exercises, often changes nothing. Medicine is sometimes a process of elimination to find a solution.

If you have a total hip or knee replacement, be aware that you will still have to work hard to bring your body back to full function, which may take as long as a year.

Too many patients seem to believe that, once the surgery's done, everything should be hunky-dory, and that a few hospital exercises will see them through.

Also, understand that passive treatment with machines, while helping to ease pain and inflammation, will do little to help your body regain strength, mobility, stability, and balance. As has been said, no one can do your push-ups for you.

Keeping your body in tip-top condition requires regular exercise and frequent movement. The latest research shows that strengthening the right muscle groups brings excellent results—so much so that people end up cancelling their scheduled surgeries, as they are no longer needed.

However, there is a right and a wrong way to do this, and you will need good guidance.

The last chapter of this book is a checklist for you and your body, so you can identify your areas of weakness and set yourself up with a way of charting your starting point and your progress.

Lasting change will not take place if you have no means of monitoring it. You will need a clear vision for your health. The mind needs a reward system to keep it focused and motivated. Ask yourself exactly what it is that you want to be able to do, whether that is playing with your grandchildren or climbing a mountain.

I've created the health scale to help you measure yourself. We are capable of becoming healthier, once we know how. So, I've included a list of books and other resources to help you on your way.

If you are feeling helpless, tell yourself that taking charge of your own health will help you ditch the victim mentality sometimes perpetuated by the health-care system.

Physical inactivity is a key cause of chronic diseases. And according to Healthline Media, headquartered in San Francisco, a review of studies over the last half-century shows physical activity reduces the risk of coronary artery disease. "The most physically active subjects generally had disease rates 50 percent lower than those who are sedentary," it noted on its website (www.healthline.com/health/heart-disease/exercise#The-Benefits-of-Exercise).

Don't overlook consistent, variable movements throughout your day, such as emptying the dishwasher, climbing stairs, and gardening.

A recent international study appears to confirm that physical activity helps prevent depression. The findings by a team at Massachusetts General Hospital (MGH) are published online in the journal *JAMA Psychiatry*.

"On average, doing more physical activity appears to protect against developing depression," says lead author Karmel Choi, PhD, of MGH's Psychiatric and Neurodevelopmental Genetics Unit. "Any activity appears to be better than none; our rough calculations suggest that replacing sitting with 15 minutes of a heart-pumping activity like running, or with an hour of moderately vigorous activity, is enough to produce the average increase in accelerometer data that was linked to a lower depression risk." An accelerometer uses body sensors to capture accurate motion data for health and medical monitoring.

Ontario sports medicine physician Jane Thornton, MD, PhD, says that if she had to pick a single thing that her patients should do to get healthier, it would be exercise. That's why she often hands her patients a different kind of prescription—one for walking.

"A whole cascade of events occurs in your body just after you start taking a few steps," the former world champion rower told the Canadian Broadcasting Corporation podcast, *The Dose*. "For many chronic conditions, walking is probably one of the best things we can do for our health."

Yes, your body is an amazing piece of machinery, provided it gets consistent tune-ups. There really are no shortcuts. Exercise is the best medicine. I am reminded of my father who, at eighty-seven, remained active and was still able to fully squat to do his gardening. He had been doing this throughout his adult life.

Problems

List your current health problems.

Solutions

List some possible solutions for your current health problems.

CHAPTER 14

Personal Health Rating Scale

I t's one thing to deal with specific health problems, but in the end, your overall physical and mental well-being count the most. So, here is a simple, general health rating scale to help you measure your cumulative progress.

Make a photocopy of the scale first, so you can do your scoring in pencil on a regular basis. This will help you keep track of your health.

Grade yourself from 1 to 10 in the twenty categories on the scale below, with 1 being the worst and 10 the best. The better your health, the higher your score. For example, scoring 10 in the Pain category signifies you are essentially pain-free; a 1 rating means you are constantly in pain. The higher your score, the better your health.

Note: In most tests, scoring is reversed. For this scale and for consistency, please use 1 for poor and 10 for great.

Circle the numbers in as honest and thoughtful a way as possible. And review them every week.

Here are the health categories in alphabetical order.

Balance

1   2   3   4   5   6   7   8   9   10

Bowel and bladder

1   2   3   4   5   6   7   8   9   10

Breathing

1   2   3   4   5   6   7   8   9   10

Career and jobs

1   2   3   4   5   6   7   8   9   10

Exercise

1   2   3   4   5   6   7   8   9   10

Family

1   2   3   4   5   6   7   8   9   10

Finances

1   2   3   4   5   6   7   8   9   10

Friendship

1   2   3   4   5   6   7   8   9   10

Happiness

1   2   3   4   5   6   7   8   9   10

Hobbies and passions

1   2   3   4   5   6   7   8   9   10

Lifestyle and medication

1 2 3 4 5 6 7 8 9 10

Marriage, single, divorced or widowed

1 2 3 4 5 6 7 8 9 10

Mobility

1 2 3 4 5 6 7 8 9 10

Pain (make sure you rate 1 as bad pain and 10 as no pain)

1 2 3 4 5 6 7 8 9 10

Relaxation

1 2 3 4 5 6 7 8 9 10

Sleep

1 2 3 4 5 6 7 8 9 10

Smoking

1 2 3 4 5 6 7 8 9 10

Strength

1 2 3 4 5 6 7 8 9 10

Stress and anxiety

1 2 3 4 5 6 7 8 9 10

Weight, diet, and digestion

1 2 3 4 5 6 7 8 9 10

During this rating process, you should be able to pinpoint which aspects of your life need attention. Pick two categories you want to work on first and decide why.

Keep your *Self-Health Fix* test handy. Don't underestimate small changes; they will become your first steps in taking control of your health. The important thing is to remain disciplined and optimistic.

I took the test recently, and quickly discovered where I was weak, namely in my ability to get a good night's sleep and in my stress level.

In total, I scored 152 points out of a possible 200 = 76%, so there is room for improvement, and I know the areas I need to work on.

To calculate your percentage, divide your total score by 2. That equals your percentage.

As a rough guide, an aggregate rating of 50% or below means your health needs attention. A rating of 50% to 75% calls for improvement. A rating of 75% to 90% is good, and 90% to 100% is excellent.

Tips for Your Self-Health Fix

Here are some tips on how to improve your scores, along with some Helpful Resources. All the recommended books are available through Amazon.

Balance

○ Challenge your balance daily by going up and down hills and walking on uneven surfaces.

○ Climb steps regularly.

○ Practise standing on one leg to put your pants on.

○ Learn to sit down and stand up slowly in your chair by using your legs, with minimal help from your hands.

○ Do foot and ankle exercises daily.

Helpful Resource

The Posture Pain Fix by physiotherapist Rosalind Ferry.

Vestibular Disorder Association VeDA (https://vestibular.org/)

Bowel and Bladder

○ Understand that this is a common problem for men and women, and you will need help sorting it out.

○ Some physiotherapists specialize in pelvic-floor problems and can provide relief through exercise, manual techniques, proper breathing, and education.

○ Specific strengthening and/or relaxation of your pelvic-floor muscles is very effective.

○ Learn how to use your body as a unit and remain balanced over your feet, pelvis, shoulders, and head.

○ Certain foods and drinks can increase your bladder sensitivity.

Helpful Resources

Ending Female Pain by Isa Herrera, MSPT

Ending Male Pelvic Pain by Isa Herrera, MSPT

Heal Pelvic Pain by Amy Stein, MPT

Healthline at www.healthline.com/health/overactive-bladder

Breathing

○ Observe your breathing patterns by placing your hands quietly on your upper chest, then moving them to your belly.

○ Reduce any tension you feel by letting go in your neck, jaw, shoulders, torso, and/or back.

○ Breathe in and out slowly through your nose and mouth, as if you were inhaling your future and exhaling your past.

○ Sit tall with an open, relaxed torso. Do not slump, as this compresses your organs and makes it harder for you to use your diaphragm and intercostal muscles to breathe optimally.

❍ Boost your breathing by laughing, singing, and exercising.

Helpful Resource

Breath: The New Science of a Lost Art by James Nestor

Career and Jobs

❍ Everybody deserves to feel valued at work, whether employed or self-employed. But so often we feel either trapped or bored. It's time to dig ourselves out of the rut.

❍ Try doing something every day, however small, to further your career.

❍ Be honest about your work limitations, but read widely about job opportunities.

❍ If you really feel you are a round peg in a square hole, be brave, seek other work, and turn your life around.

❍ Seek the help of a career coach or mentor.

Helpful Resource

Designing Your Life by Bill Burnett and Dave Evans

Your Simplest Life by Lisa Turner

Exercise

❍ Make an honest assessment about your fitness level regularly, using the Personal Health Rating Scale.

○ Decide what it is you want to be able to do, whether it's strolling along the beach or running a marathon.

○ Try to set aside a time to exercise. And don't leave it until the last thing in the day.

○ Find a friend with whom to walk, dance, or play tennis. You will help each other remain focused and committed.

○ The more you exercise, the better you will feel, function, and sleep.

○ Lifting weights or doing other resistance training improves your bone density and overall health.

○ Get 15 to 20 minutes of sun daily to help your body make natural Vitamin D. This helps serotonin, the hormone that makes you feel good.

Helpful Resources

Your Body's Many Cries for Water by F. Batmanghelidj, MD

The Core Program by Peggy W. Brill, PT

Strength Training Over 40 by Alana Collins

Stretching to Stay Young by Jessica Matthews

"6-Minute Fitness at 60+" by Dr. Jonathan Su, DPT

Urbanpoling.com for Activator Rehab Poles for improving your walking, core and posture.

Family

○ The members of your family can be a great source of strength. Don't be afraid to embrace that source.

○ Family problems can also be debilitating. So, sort them out as quickly as possible.

○ Learn about setting boundaries for yourself and others.

○ Learn how to bless and release . . . and to have fun and live lightly.

○ Families that play together tend to stay together.

Helpful Resource

It Didn't Start with You by Mark Wolynn

Finances

○ Ease your money worries by finding ways to pay down any debt.

○ Improve your attitude to money by reading deeply and widely about financial matters.

○ If need be, seek debt or financial counselling.

○ If you can, save 10 percent of whatever money you bring in. Let it accumulate. That is your nest egg, your reserve fund.

○ Money is energy, so keep it circulating. Believe you deserve to have it.

Helpful Resources

Happy Money by Ken Honda

The Psychology of Money by Morgan Housel

Friendship

○ Socializing is key to our health. Try joining a group or initiating small talk with friends, relatives, and neighbours.

○ If you feel lonely, don't let your feelings fester. Help yourself by giving to others and becoming a volunteer.

○ Try a meditation class or join a local sports team.

○ Sign up for a book club or writing group.

○ Spend time with a pet or other furry friend.

○ Help out at the local pet shelter.

Helpful Resource

The Charisma Myth by Olivia Fox Cabane

Happiness

○ Realize it's unrealistic for humans to be happy all the time. But you should prize happiness.

○ Be a positive, drama-free person. Don't let other people get you down; misery attracts misery.

○ Smile, stand tall, and open your chest. This tells your brain you feel confident and ready to tackle the world.

○ Happy people attract other happy people.

Helpful resource

The Happiness Project by Gretchen Rubin

The Happiness Advantage by Shawn Achor

Hobbies and Passions

○ Develop your passions and hobbies, whether dancing, fishing, gardening, golfing, hiking, painting, stamp collecting, or skydiving.

○ If you don't have something you feel passionate about, look back to your childhood and see what got you excited then. Try it out now.

○ Take the time to explore what raises your curiosity or interest. You have only one life, so live it to the fullest.

○ Work your body, but also prime your mind. Don't ignore the little pleasures, such as playing scrabble or doing crosswords.

Helpful Resource

How to Find Your Passion by Michelle Kulp

Lifestyle and Medication

○ If you are taking medications, talk with your doctor and/or pharmacist about the pills you are taking and see whether they can be safely reduced.

❍ Prescription drugs often have side-effects, which may be causing some of your problems.

❍ Sleeping pills can be highly addictive and detrimental to your health. Withdraw from them very slowly and only with medical guidance.

❍ Check with your doctor to see whether you can make lifestyle changes to avoid the need for medication.

❍ Movement and exercise are often the best medication. So are sunshine and fresh air.

Helpful Resource

The Side Effects Bible by Frederic Vagnini, MD, and Barry Fox, PhD

Married, Single, Divorced, or Widowed

❍ Work consistently on your marriage as it's an important part of your overall health.

❍ Listen to and otherwise make time for your partner. If need be, enlist the help of a counselor.

❍ Go out regularly and have fun together with free-flowing conversation.

❍ Stop criticizing your mate, but focus instead on what makes him or her happy.

❍ If you are single and struggling, learn to be happy with yourself first.

❍ If you are mourning the loss of your soulmate or friend ...I am so sorry. Find a counselor and relatable resources to help you through your grief.

Helpful Resource

Quantum Love by Laura Berman, PhD

It's OK that You're Not OK by Megan Devine

Single on Purpose by John Kim

The Gifts of Imperfection by Brené Brown

Mobility

❍ Start by doing some easy walking or other simple movements to lubricate your joints.

❍ Increase your flexibility, muscle strength, and balance through day-to-day activities.

❍ Consider reviewing your diet to reduce inflammation in your body. You may need professional help here.

❍ The more you do, the more you'll do. The opposite is also true.

❍ Give yourself small, daily, achievable goals.

Helpful Resources

Instant Relief by Peggy W. Brill, PT

Stretching to Stay Young by Jessica Matthews

Urbanpoling.com Activator Rehab Poles

The Foot Fix by Yamuna Zake

Pain

❍ Do you have acute or long-term pain? Each one will require a different approach.

❍ What steps have you taken to control your pain? Medication, physiotherapy, massage, chiropractic, and so on?

❍ Pain is a protector, but it can itself become a disease. Fear of movement because of pain can delay your recovery.

❍ If you are in a lot of pain, focus on what you can do and gradually do more. Distractions can help redirect your brain away from pain.

❍ Try using breathing exercises and other relaxation techniques to ease your pain.

❍ Try Epsom Salts baths or a foot soak for 20 minutes. Magnesium in the salts is important for relaxation and nerve and muscle function. Check with your doctor or pharmacist before use.

❍ Your skin might itch or tingle after the bath if you are low in magnesium.

Helpful Resources

Joette Calabrese, Practical Homeopathy at joettecalabrese.com

Donna Eden, Eden Method at edenenergymedicine.com

Pain Free by Pete Egoscue

Bye-Bye Back Pain by Dr. Grace Walker Gray

The Tapping Solution for Pain Relief by Nick Ortner

Awareness Heals by Steven Shafarman

Tamethebeast.org for chronic pain

Relaxation

- ○ Focus on what you do for relaxation. Is it enough or should you try for more?
- ○ Engage in sports and other forms of exercise to help you lead a relaxed life.
- ○ Learn how to breathe better through meditation, yoga, tai chi, qi gong, or other body awareness disciplines.
- ○ Music, drawing, reading, colouring, knitting, and other crafts are more relaxing than you might think.
- ○ Socializing is soothing.

Helpful Resources

The Relaxation and Stress Reduction Workbook by Martha Davis

Lee Holden, Qi Gong Master at holdenqigong.com

Sleep

- ○ Get up at the same time every morning. To calculate your bedtime, count backwards seven to eight hours from your rising time.
- ○ Try going to bed half an hour earlier to help reset your bedtime.

○ Stop eating and drinking three hours before bedtime.

○ Don't have any caffeinated drinks or chocolate after 2:00 p.m., as these are stimulants and will disturb your sleep.

○ Check thesleepdoctor.com for relevant blog posts.

○ Don't do any computer work two hours before bed. Even your device's low-light mode emits the blue light that affects the sleep hormone melatonin.

○ Blue-light filter glasses (available through Amazon or thesleepdoctor.com) can also help.

○ To assist your sleep cycle, try getting at least 15 minutes of daylight exposure in the morning and an hour of relaxation before bed.

Helpful Resource

Sleep It Off by Stella Loichot

Smoking

○ Smoking is a notoriously hard addiction to overcome. So, find a good reason to do so.

○ Think of the impact your smoking is having on your family and friends.

○ Try hypnosis to help you quit.

○ When you have an urge to smoke, drink some water instead.

○ Learn breathing techniques to help master your stress and boost your willpower.

○ Seek professional help.

Helpful Resource

The Easy Way to Stop Smoking by Allen Carr

Strength

○ Pinpoint where you score low and focus on strengthening those areas.

○ Learn how to build muscles through specific targeted exercises.

○ Enlist the help of a fitness professional to show you how to do your exercises correctly.

○ Use everything from hand weights to resistance bands to tone your upper and lower body.

○ Do squats, starting with 10 and building up to 30 repetitions.

○ Gardening, skiing, and other outdoor pursuits are natural strength builders.

Helpful Resource

Bigger Leaner Stronger by Michael Matthews

The Year One Challenge for Women by Michael Matthews

Stress and Anxiety

○ Identify the source of your stress, whether from your job, marriage, family, finances, or health.

○ Tackle one or two of the above stress sources.

○ Try stress-reducing meditation and breathing exercises.

○ Seek a counselor for your stress.

○ Examine whether your anxiety is connected to a particular time or specific event in your life.

○ Consider whether your anxiety is the result of ongoing gut issues. Have you had a concussion or PTSD? Either of these conditions can alter brain messaging to the gut.

○ Deep-breathing exercises can help you activate your parasympathetic (rest and digest) and deactivate sympathetic (fight or flight) nervous systems, calming you and your nervous system.

Helpful Resources

Joette Calabrese, Practical Homeopathy at joettecalabrese.com

The Little Book of Mindfulness by Dr. Patrizia Collar

The Tapping Solution by Nick Ortner and Mark Hyman

The Antianxiety Food Solution by Trudy Scott, CN

Weight, Diet, and Digestion

○ Write down daily what you eat. Reduce or cut out candies, cookies, and other sugary foods.

○ Talk to a dietician about improving your diet, especially if you have inflammation.

○ Reduce your consumption of alcoholic drinks, pop, fruit juices and diet sodas.

○ Make sure you get a good night's sleep. Poor sleep can really affect your weight.

○ Taking antibiotics will seriously affect your gut health and digestion.

○ Increase your activity level, and walk and move with purpose.

○ Being overweight stresses your joints and contributes to wear and tear in your hips, knees, and other joints.

○ Drink water regularly throughout your day.

Helpful Resources

Joette Calabrese, Practical Homeopathy at joettecalabrese.com

The Obesity Code by Jason Fung

GI Society at badgut.org

GLA:D™ Canada program at gladcanada.ca for people with hip and knee osteoarthritis

The Plant Paradox by Steven R. Gundry

Activate Your Vagus Nerve by Dr. Navaz Habib

Mayo Clinic at mayoclinic.org

Author

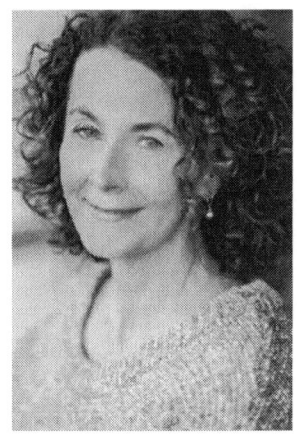

Rosalind Ferry is a long-time British Columbia physiotherapist, author of the book *The Posture Pain Fix* and co-author (nine authors) of *Shine, Volume 3: Inspirational Stories of Choosing Success Over Adversity* (Prominence Publishing, 2019). Over the years, she has helped thousands of people with every kind of condition: sore necks, bad backs, wonky knees, balance and dizziness disorders, and trauma.

Her patients have included everyone from young soccer players with sports injuries to senior citizens with mobility issues. They have told her they appreciate her calmness, common sense, willingness to listen, and holistic approach to their treatment.

Her inspiration has come from her love of horses, animals, and the great outdoors, plus her enjoyment in seeing others succeed in dealing with their pain and regaining control over their lives.

Her own struggle with chronic ear and hearing problems has made her empathize fully with those battling similarly debilitating, complex problems.

Her philosophy has been one of combining physical treatment with an appreciation of the parts that stress and other psychological issues play in patients' overall health. She puts her trust in the Latin maxim: *Mens sana in corpore sano*, "a healthy mind in a healthy body."

Manufactured by Amazon.ca
Bolton, ON